T0406051

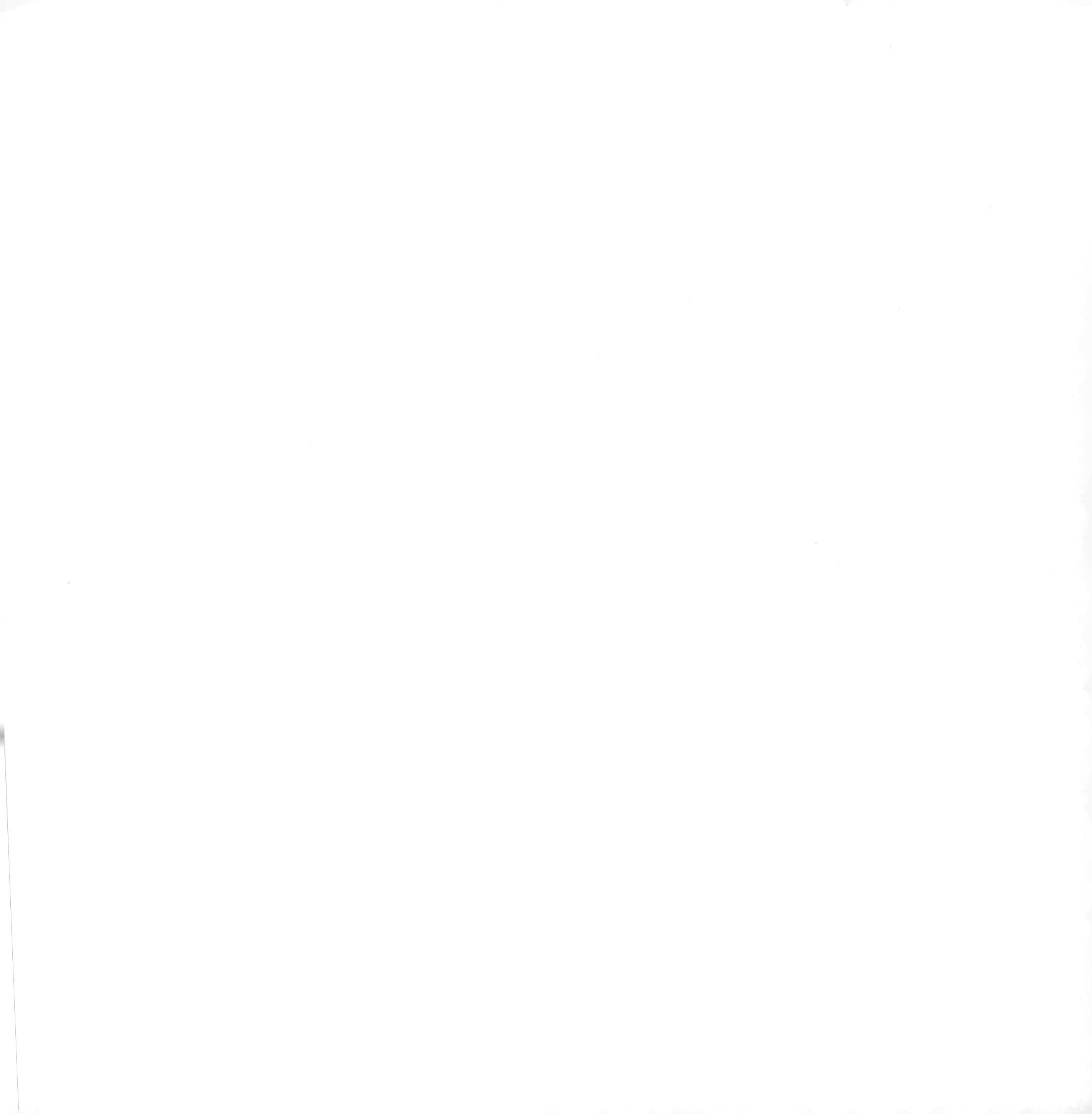

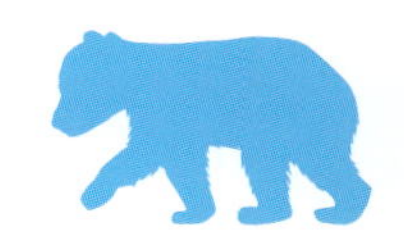

FART

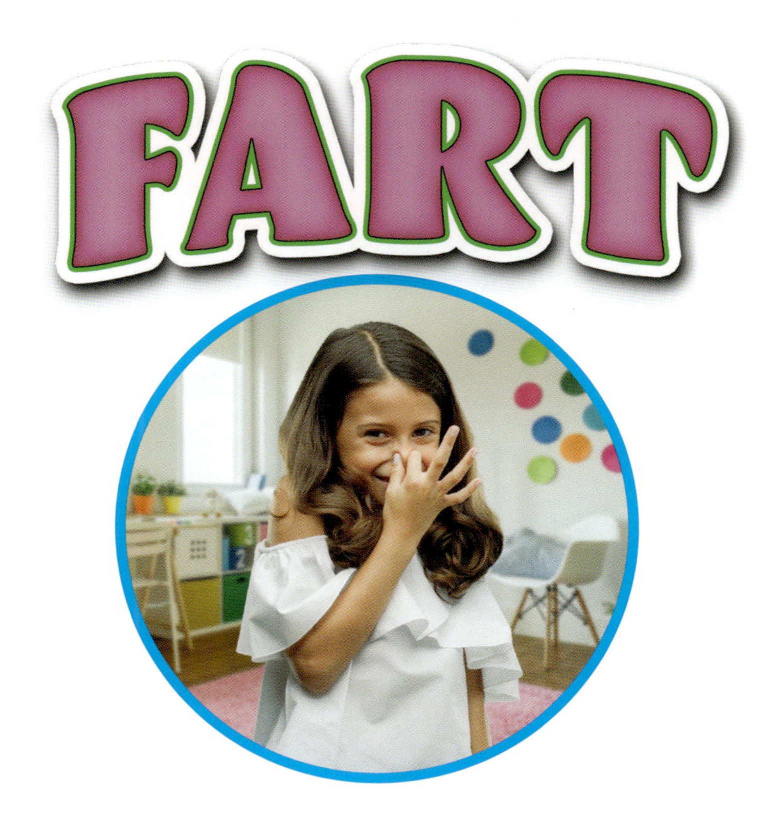

by Rachel Rose

Consultant: Beth Gambro
Reading Specialist, Yorkville, Illinois

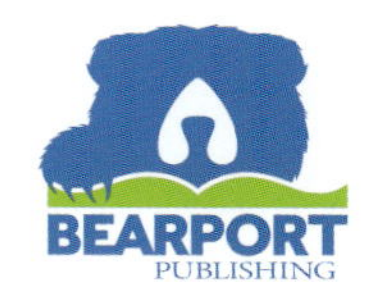

Minneapolis, Minnesota

Teaching Tips

Before Reading

- Look at the cover of the book. Discuss the picture and the title.
- Ask readers to brainstorm a list of what they already know about farts. What can they expect to see in this book?
- Go on a picture walk, looking through the pictures to discuss vocabulary and make predictions about the text.

During Reading

- Read for purpose. Encourage readers to think about farts as they are reading.
- Ask readers to look for the details of the book. What are they learning about the body and how it makes farts?
- If readers encounter an unknown word, ask them to look at the sounds in the word. Then, ask them to look at the rest of the page. Are there any clues to help them understand?

After Reading

- Encourage readers to pick a buddy and reread the book together.
- Ask readers to describe what can make some farts stinky. Find the page that tells about stinky farts.
- Ask readers to write or draw something they learned about farts.

Credits: Cover and title page, © AaronAmat/iStock and © Photographee.eu/Shutterstock; 5, © Aleksandra Suzi/Shutterstock; 6, © PavelHlystov/iStock; 7, © FatCamera/iStock; 8–9, © PeopleImages/iStock; 11, © aleks333/Shutterstock; 12–13, © Jihan Nafiaa Zahri/Shutterstock; 15, © Susanne Kischnick/iStock; 16–17, © WAYHOME studio/Shutterstock and © Valeriya/iStock; 18, © FatCamera/iStock; 20–21, © PeopleImages/iStock; 22, © Tetiana Lazunova/iStock; 23TL, © Hakase_/iStock; 23TR, © ShantiHesse/iStock; 23BL, © Hakase_/iStock; and 23BR, © yodiyim/iStock.

Library of Congress Cataloging-in-Publication Data is available at www.loc.gov or upon request from the publisher.

ISBN: 978-1-63691-819-8 (hardcover)
ISBN: 978-1-63691-826-6 (paperback)
ISBN: 978-1-63691-833-4 (ebook)

For more information, write to Bearport Publishing, 5357 Penn Avenue South, Minneapolis, MN 55419. Printed in the United States of America.

Contents

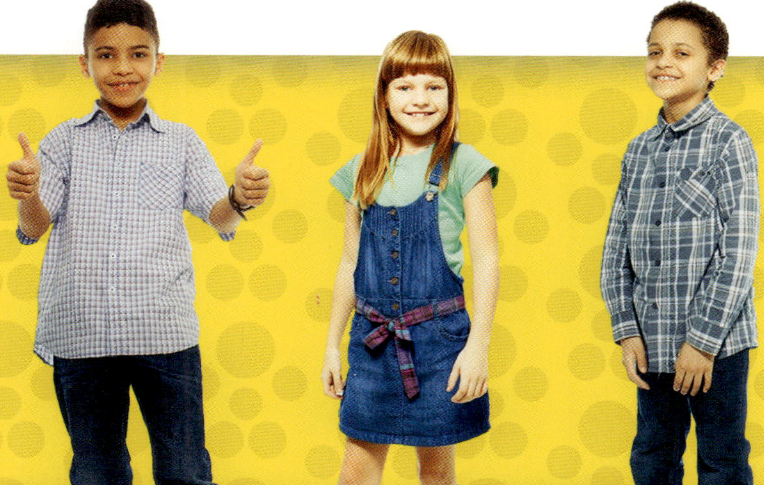

What Is That Smell?

I had a yummy lunch.

But now my tummy feels funny.

Pfft!

Why does my body do that?

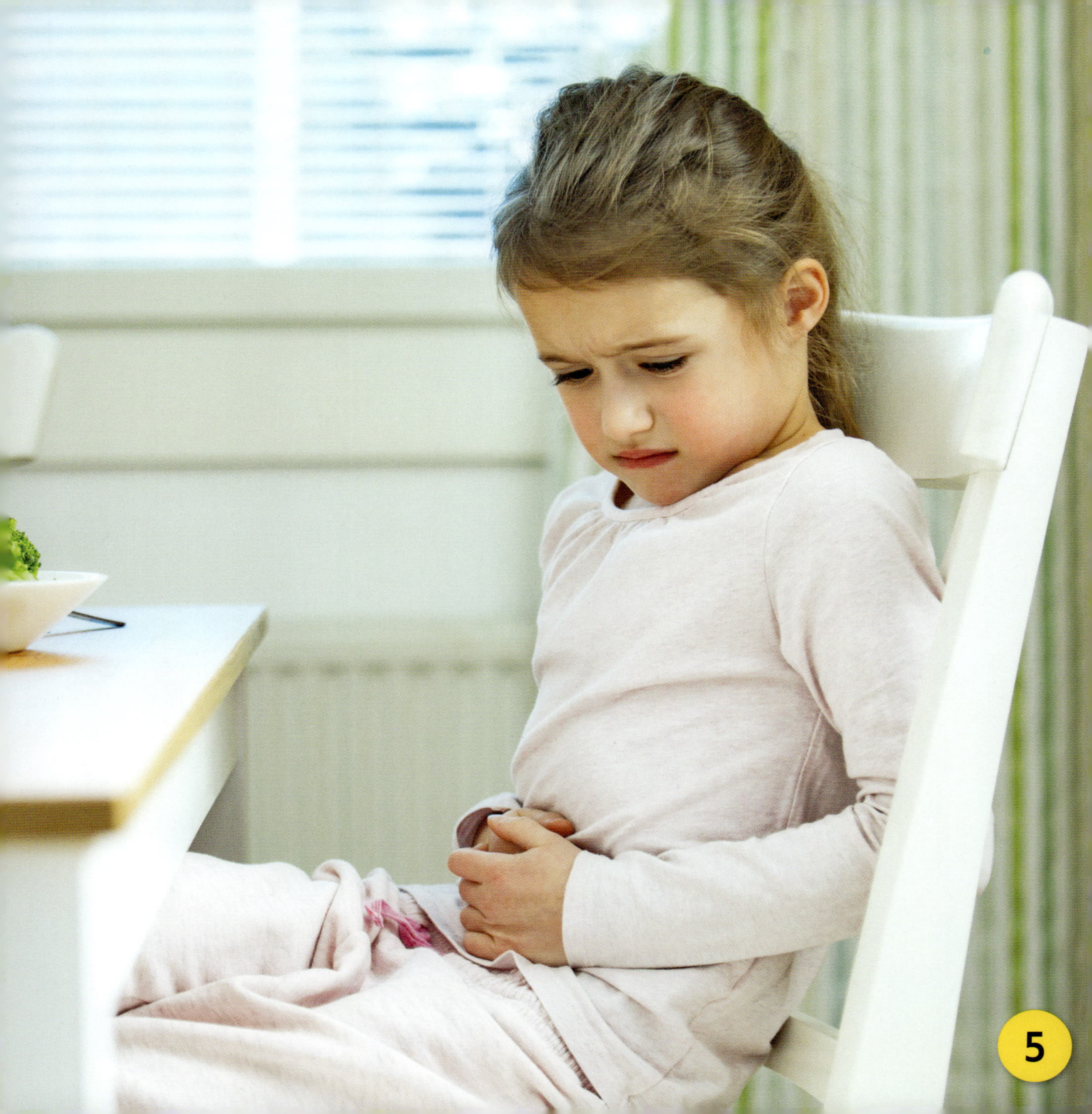

Everybody farts.

Your family and friends fart.

And you do, too!

But how do farts happen?

It all starts after you eat.

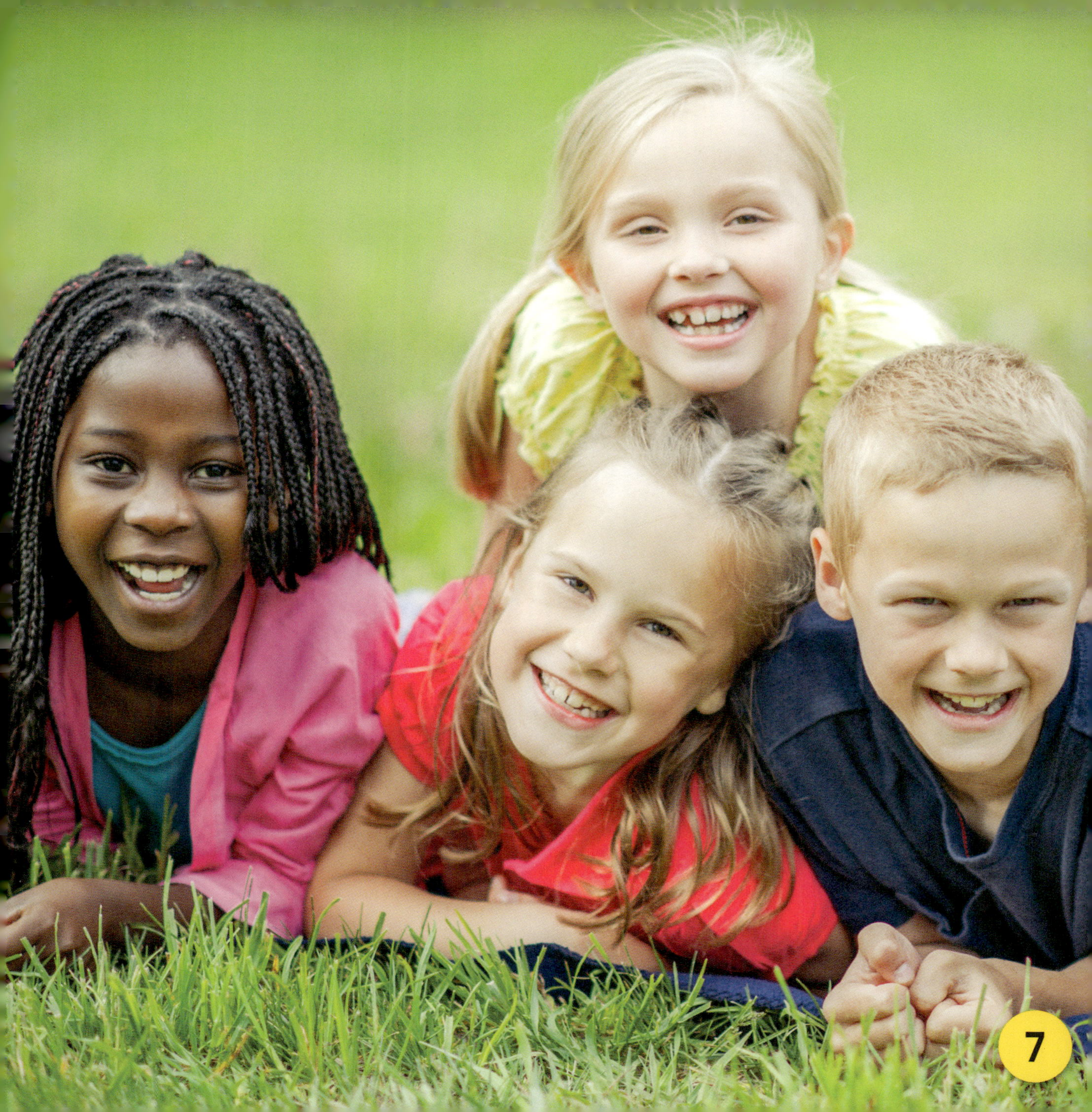

Food goes from your mouth to your **stomach**.

Then, your body starts to break down the food.

That makes **gases**.

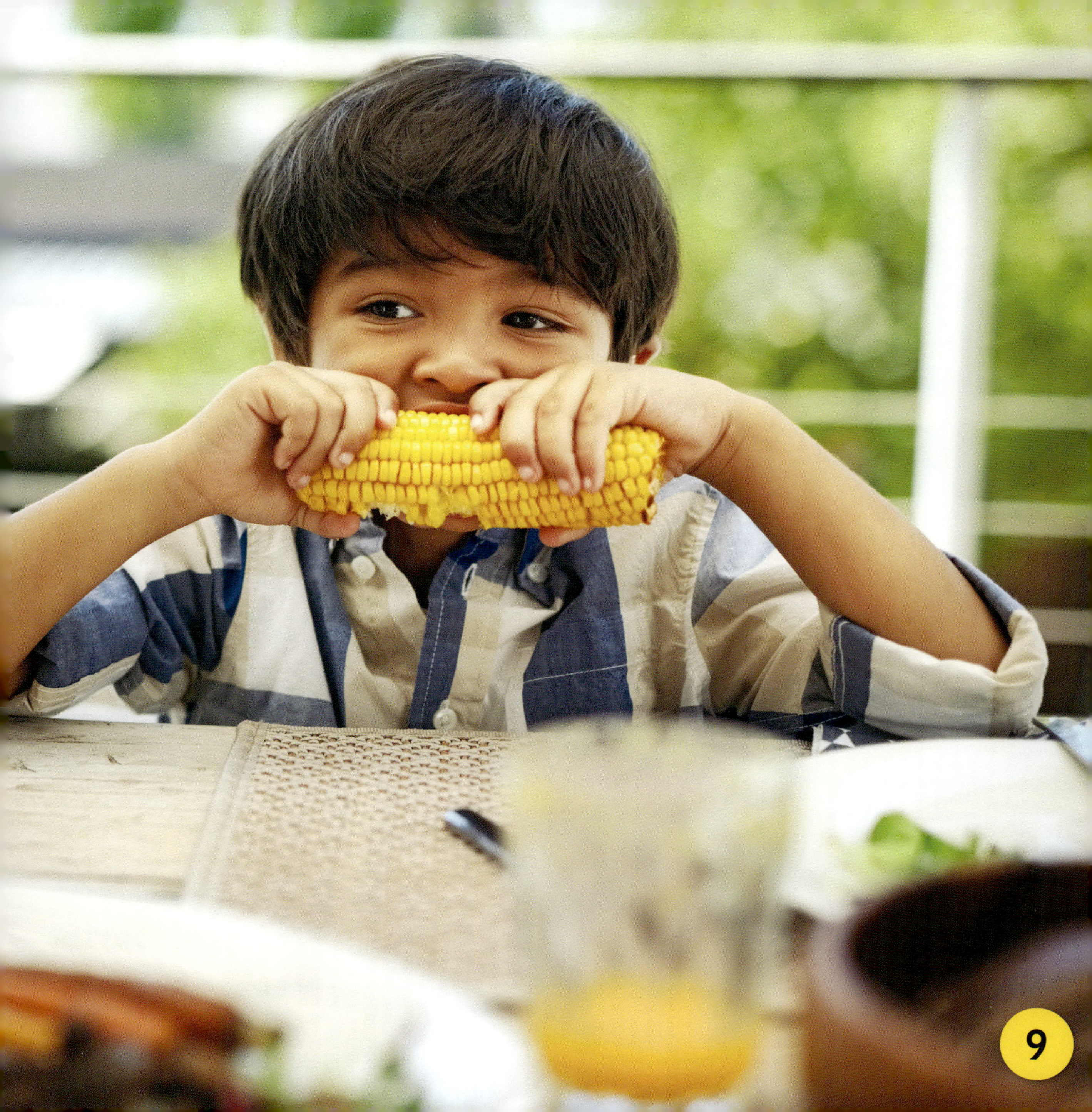

The gases need to leave your body somehow.

One way out is through your bottom.

Gases come out as farts.

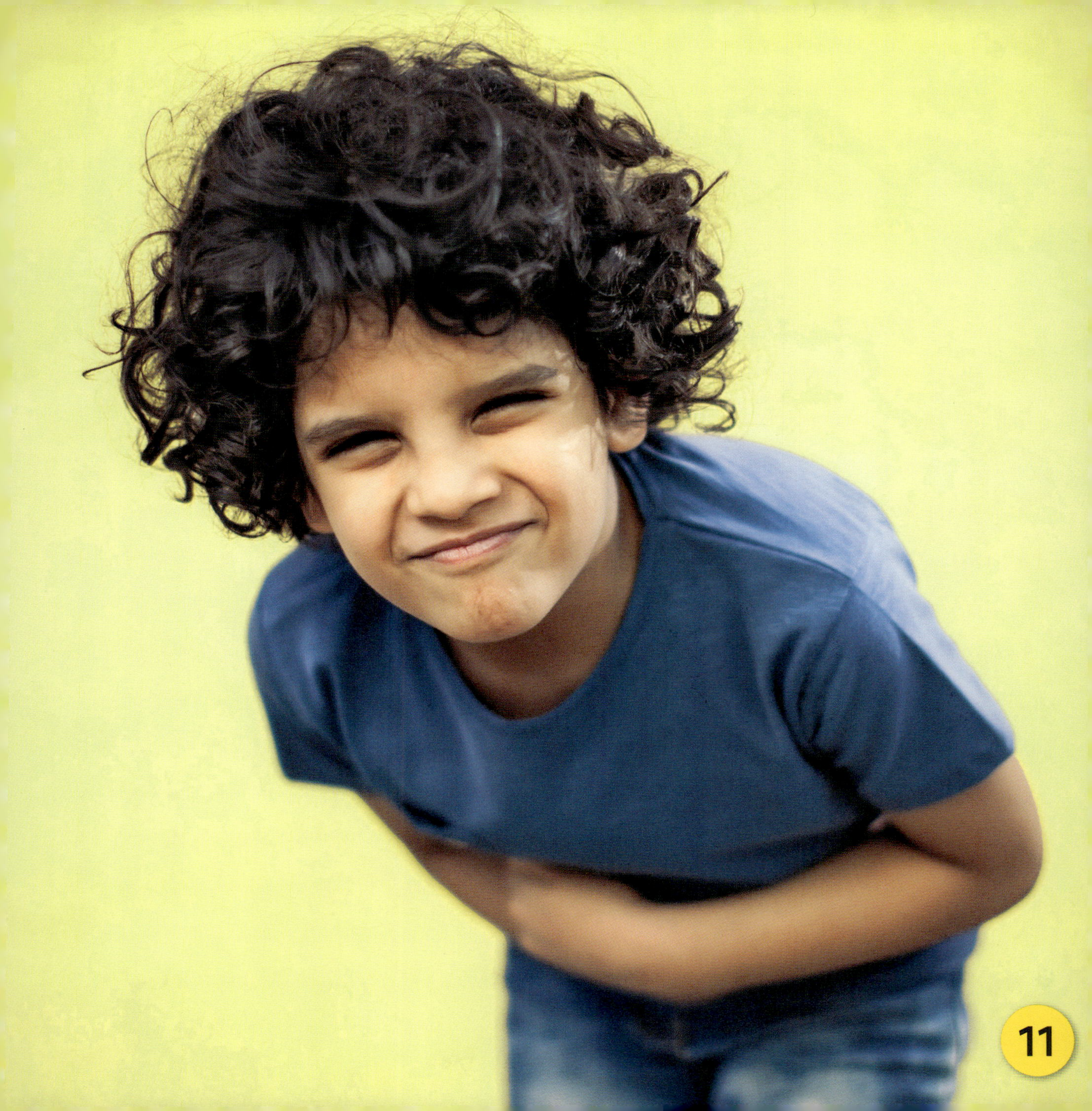

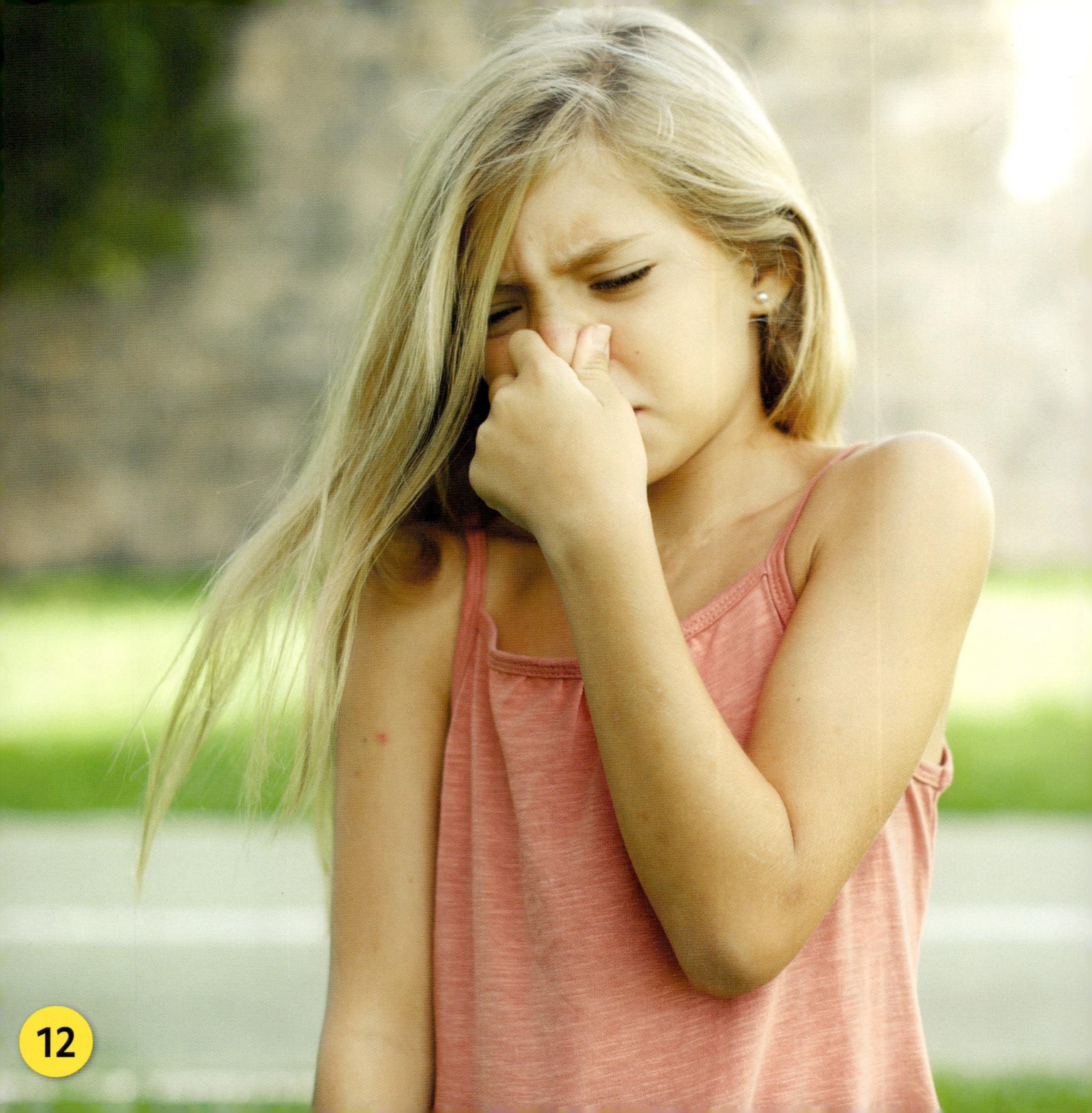

Sometimes, farts
make sounds.

But mostly they
are quiet.

Some farts smell bad.

Pee-yew!

Often, they do not
smell at all!

Why are some farts stinky?

Some foods are more work for your stomach to break down.

The gases from these foods can smell bad.

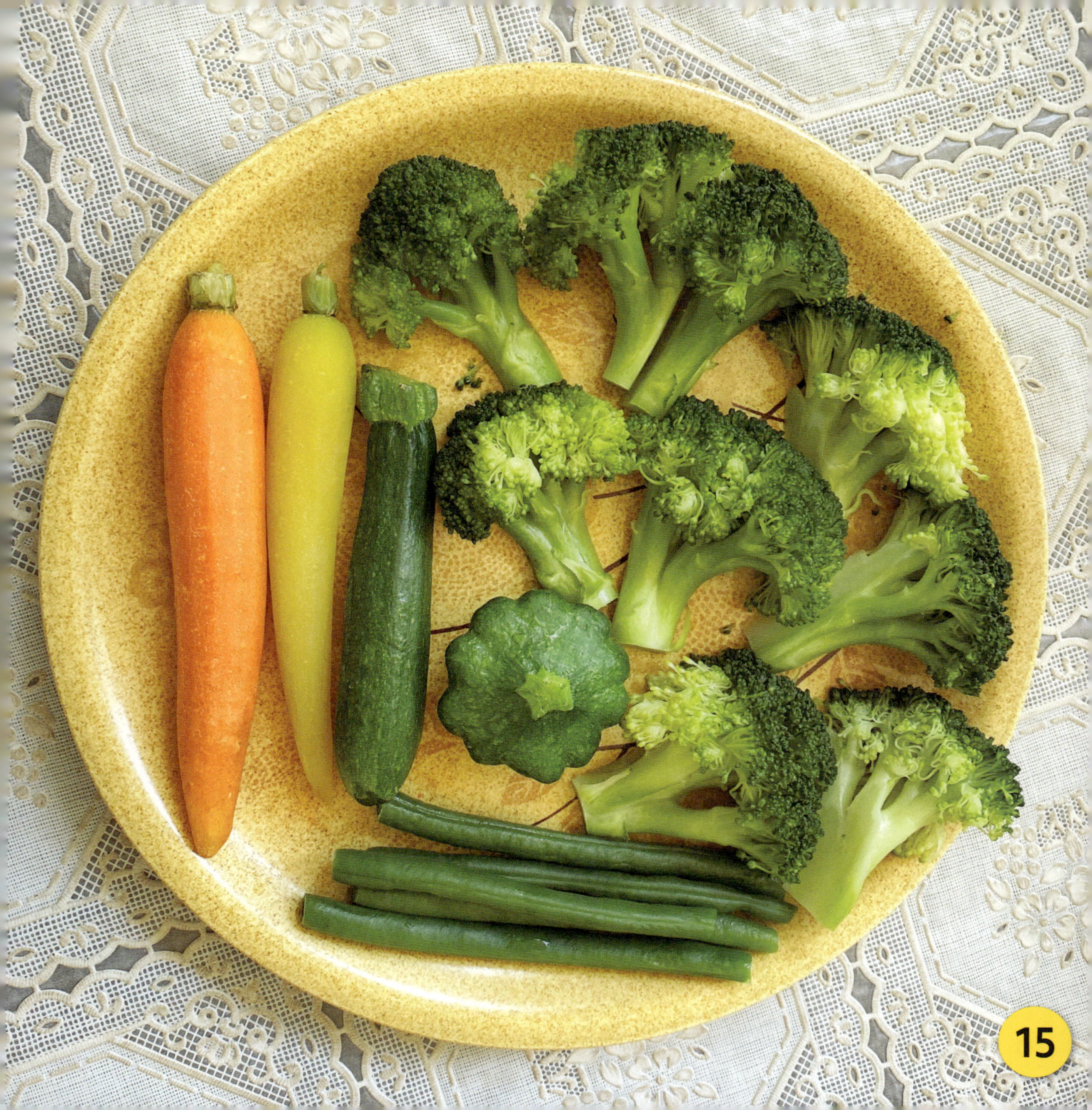

You can also fart after you **breathe** in extra air.

These kinds of farts do not smell.

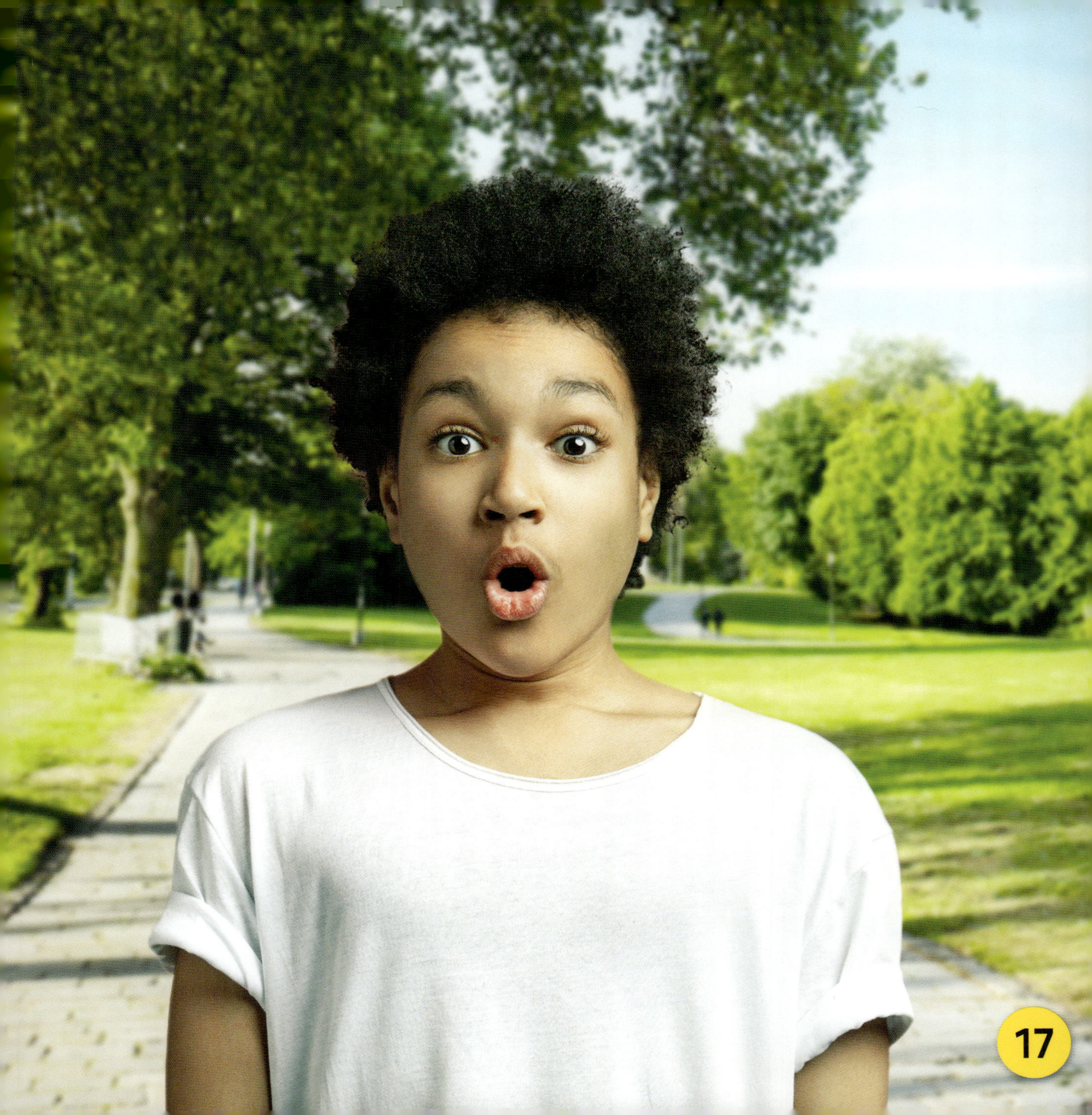

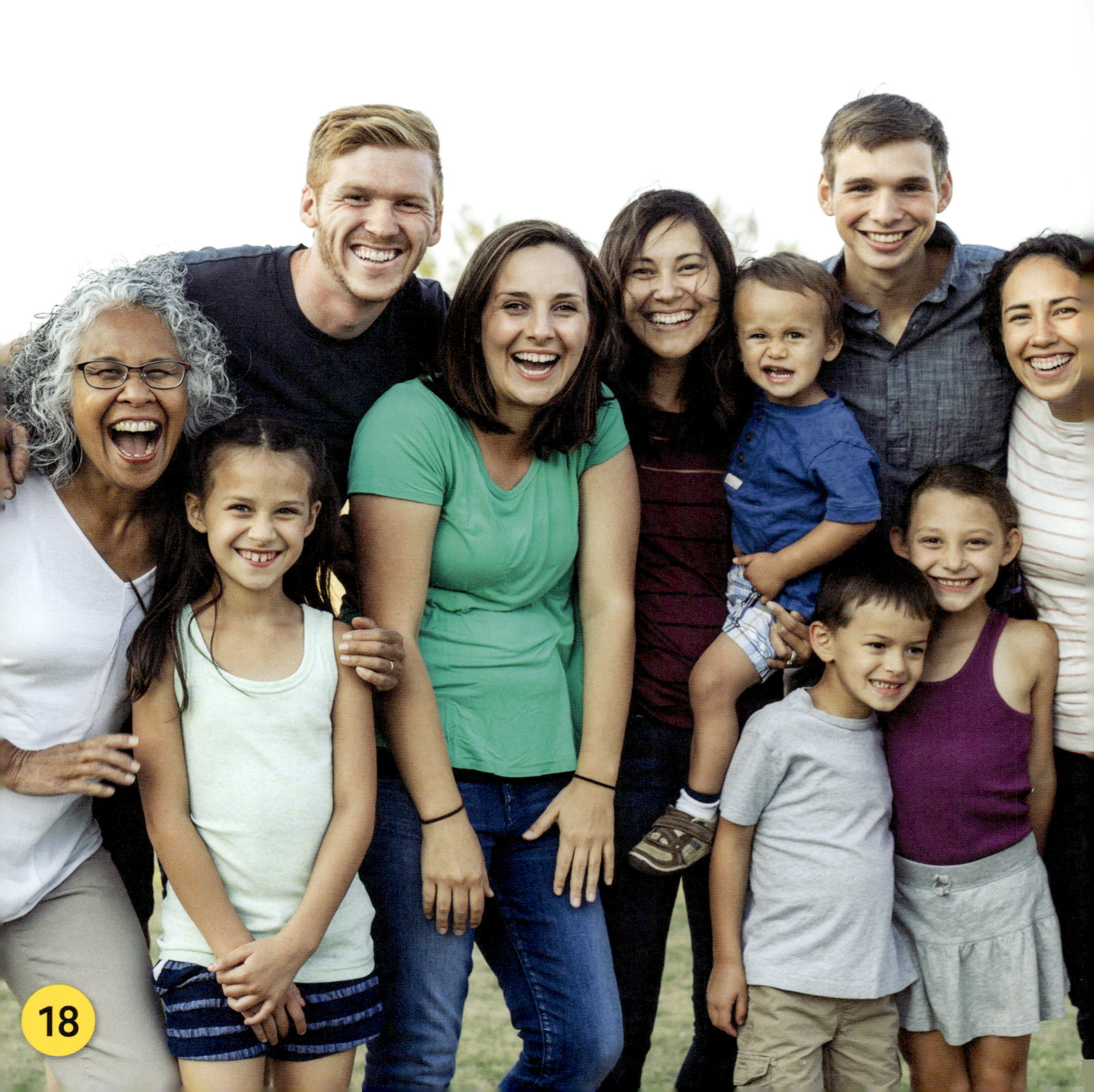

You should not try to stop farts.

They help keep your body **healthy**.

It is okay to fart.

Remember, everybody does it!

People fart more often than you might think.

Everybody farts at least 10 times a day!

How many times did you fart today?

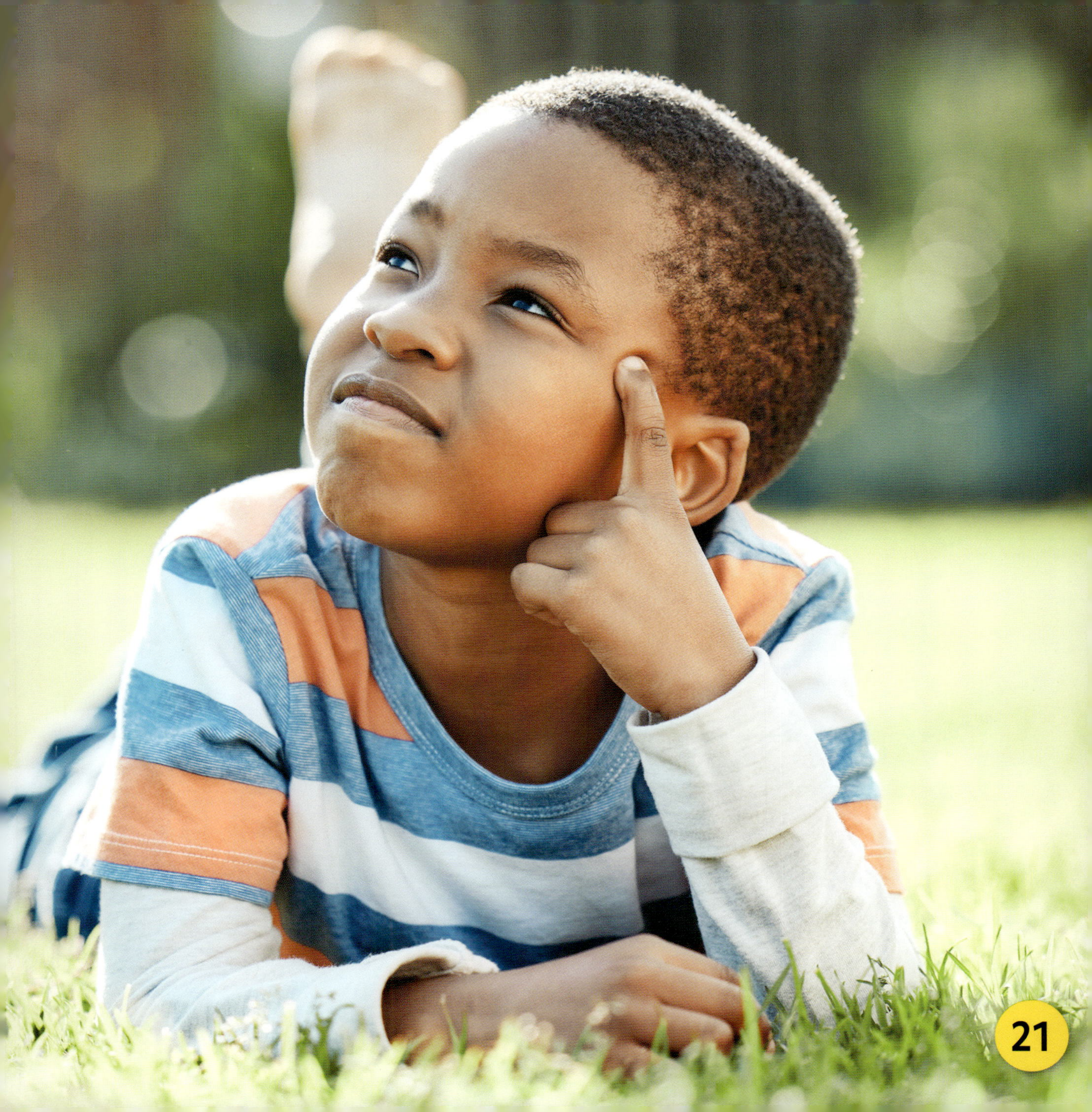

See It Happen

You eat food.

The food goes to your stomach.

As food in the stomach is broken down, gases form.

The gases leave through your bottom.

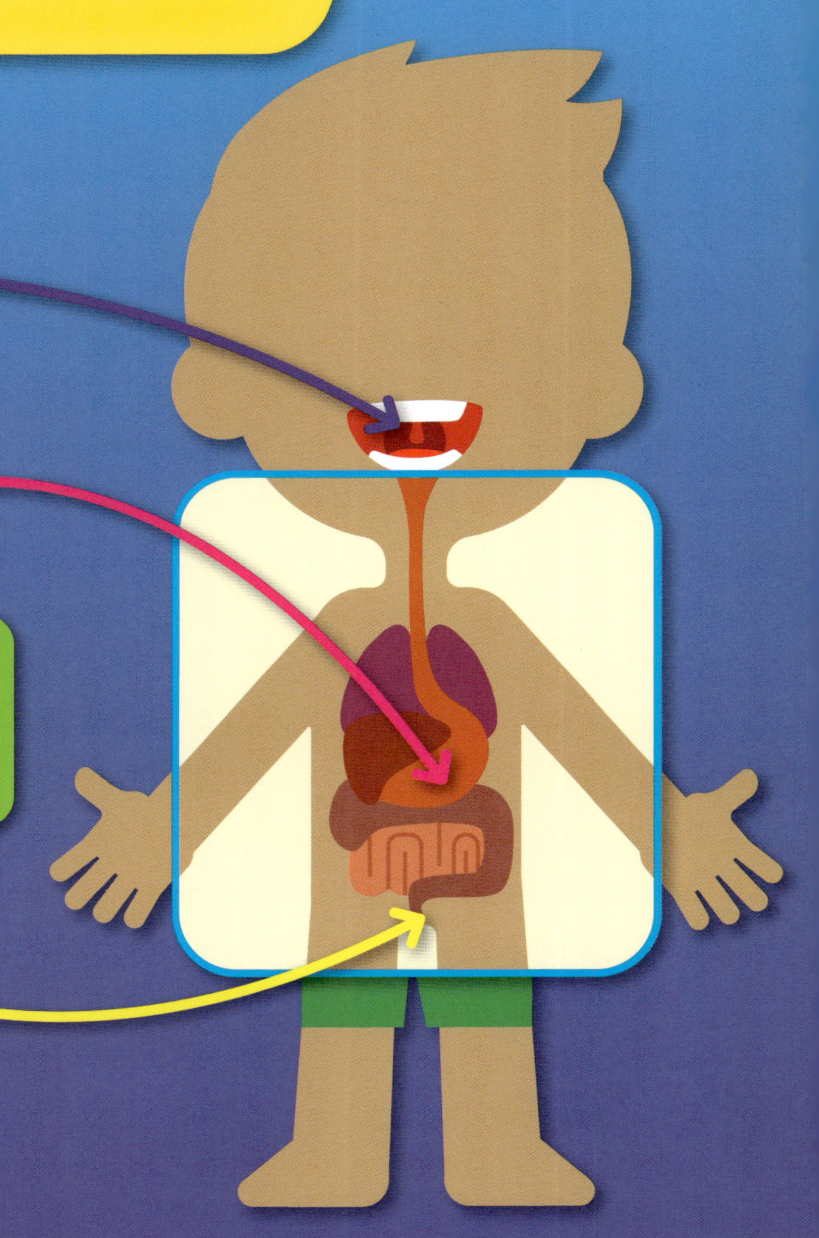

Glossary

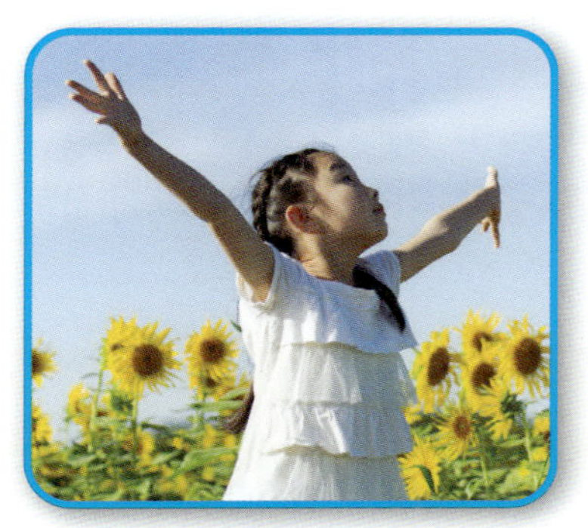

breathe to take air in and let it out of the body

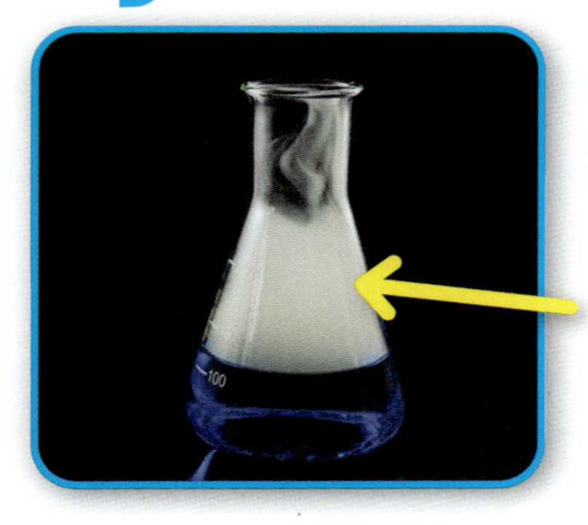

gases things like air with no shape

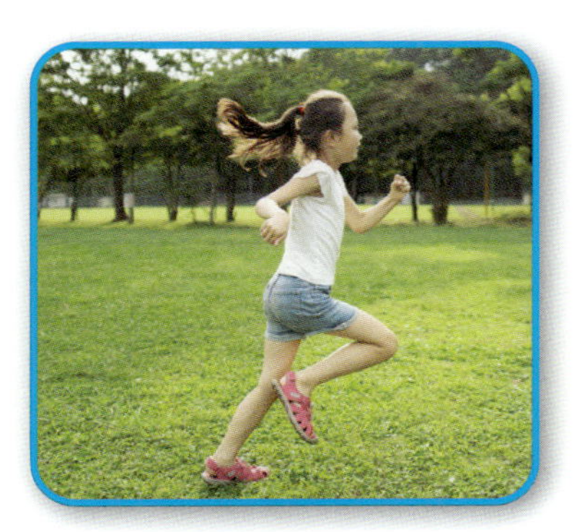

healthy not ill

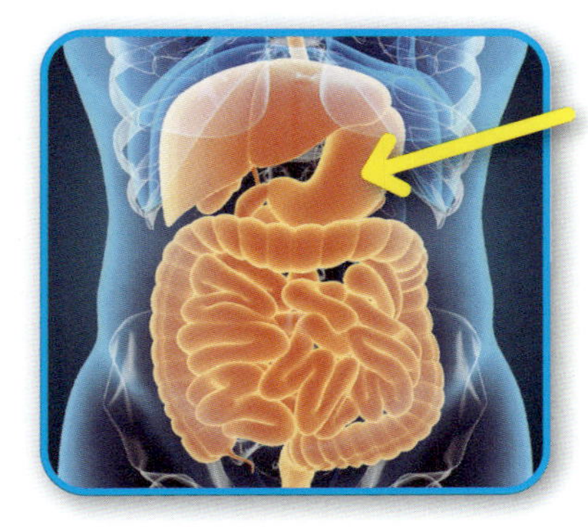

stomach the part of the body that breaks down food

Index

Read More

Hansen, Grace. *Farts (Beginning Science: Gross Body Functions).* Minneapolis: Abdo Kids, 2020.

Hughes, Sloane. *My Stomach (What's Inside Me?).* Minneapolis: Bearport Publishing Company, 2022.

Learn More Online

1. Go to **www.factsurfer.com** or scan the QR code below.
2. Enter "**Fart**" into the search box.
3. Click on the cover of this book to see a list of websites.

About the Author

Rachel Rose lives in California. She can't believe people fart as much as they do!